Sustainable Fitness

Protecting the Planet While Improving Your Health

Table of Contents

Chapter 1. Introduction

Introducing a groundbreaking Special Report that harmoniously ties in the health of our planet and individual fitness like never before: "Sustainable Fitness: Protecting the Planet While Improving Your Health". As we sculpt a healthier, fitter version of ourselves, shouldn't we also aim to preserve the planet that we call home? This empowering report not only motivates you to be in the best physical shape but also champions eco-friendly habits. Bonded beautifully by fascinating stories, real-life case studies, and leading industry insights, this sustainability-meets-fitness report forms an intricate and invigorating read. If you're eager to embark on a fitness journey that sings the song of sustainability, this Special Report is your perfect companion. Prepare to be inspired, educated, and moved into action. Buy your copy now to help make your personal fitness voyage part of the larger journey toward a healthier, greener world!

Chapter 2. Redefining Fitness: A New Outlook

Traditionally, when we imagine fitness, our minds often envision rippling muscles, lean physiques, and high-energy workouts. However, the modern notion of health and wellness is undergoing a revolution, one where mindfulness, mental wellness, and planetary health are as celebrated as physical robustness.

2.1. Personal Wellbeing and Planetary Health: Two Sides of the Same Coin

In this new fitness landscape, the wellbeing of the individual and the planet are seen as intrinsically linked. As humans in the Anthropocene - the epoch of significant human impact on the planet's ecosystems - we understand the reciprocal relationship that our actions have with our surroundings. What is good for us can also be good for the Earth. However, this linkage requires us to redefine our fitness regimes and lifestyle choices to integrate sustainable practices.

Presently, we confront a dual global crisis: personal health and planetary health. Obesity rates are rising alongside greenhouse gas emissions. Instead of seeing these crises as separate, we can approach them as two sides of a coin. The resources we use for fuel (food), comfort (homes), and mobility (transport) - which largely contribute to chronic diseases like obesity and diabetes, also drive climate change.

2.2. A Paradigm Shift: Towards Sustainable Fitness

Transitioning towards 'sustainable fitness' requires a holistic approach; one that invites us to redefine fitness beyond the narrow confines of physical training and nutritional plans. It entails considering not just how we look or feel, but also our mental wellness, societal contribution, and environmental impact.

Sustainable fitness steers us towards healthier foods, which often have a lower environmental footprint; plant-based diets being the most cogent instance. It encourages active transportation such as walking or cycling, thereby reducing our carbon footprint. And, it promotes activities in nature, contributing to our mental health whilst fostering our connection with our environment.

2.3. The Magic of Movement

Adopting active modes of transportation sparks a double-win situation: personal health improvement and carbon footprint reduction. People who walk or cycle instead of driving or taking the bus save carbon emissions, keep the air clean, and boost their cardiovascular health.

Many urban areas are working towards becoming '15-minute' cities where all necessities are within a 15-minute walk or bike ride. This approach encourages active transportation, leading to healthier residents and lower greenhouse gas emissions. This way, fitness is naturally woven into our daily routine without requiring extra time or gym equipment.

2.4. Diet: Nourishing the Body and the Earth

Dietary choices have far-reaching impacts on both our personal health and the health of the planet. Foods rich in sugar and saturated fats contribute to chronic health conditions like heart disease and diabetes, while their production also emits substantial greenhouse gases.

Adopting a plant-based diet combats this issue. Not only does it provide a plethora of nutrients, it also reduces our carbon footprint since growing plants requires fewer resources than rearing animals. Even slight shifts towards eating more plant-based meals can make a drastic difference.

Reducing food waste also plays a pivotal role in a sustainable diet. Minimizing waste not only saves money but also lessens the burden on our planet's resources.

2.5. Connection to Nature: The Key to Sustainable Fitness

Finding fitness activities that strengthen our bond with nature fosters a sense of appreciation and responsibility towards the environment. Exercising in natural settings offers physical benefits whilst acting as a natural stress reliever and mood booster. This connection motivates us to partake in environmental conservation efforts, bringing us full circle to sustainable fitness.

A study by Stanford University even found that a 50-minute walk in nature significantly reduces anxiety and increases feelings of happiness compared to walking in an urban environment. Therefore, incorporating outdoor activities into our workout routine promotes a healthier mind and body while underscoring our commitment to environmental well-being.

In conclusion, sustainable fitness involves redefining our relationship with fitness activities, diet, and nature. It encourages a paradigm shift towards a healthier lifestyle that benefits both us and our environment. By making these incremental changes today, every individual's journey towards fitness can contribute to a healthier, more sustainable planet.

Chapter 3. The Role of Environmental Sustainability in Health Promotion

Understanding the intricate relationship between environmental sustainability and health promotion is pivotal to motivating action towards creating a healthier and greener world. Our individual and collective health is closely intertwined with the health of our planet.

3.1. The Interplay of Environmental Sustainability and Health

Environmental sustainability refers to responsible interaction with the environment, conserving resources, and creating equitably distributed benefits over the long term. It encompasses a broad range of activities, from resource conservation to reduction of pollutants. This forms a basis upon which we can maintain the health of our planet. Yet, environmental sustainability is not just about the planet; it significantly impacts human health and wellness.

Many environmental factors directly and indirectly influence human health. These range from the quality of the air we breathe, the food we eat, to the communities in which we live. Impurity-laden air, for instance, can lead to respiratory diseases such as asthma. Again, polluted rivers and oceans result in tainted seafood, exposing humans to harmful toxins.

Conversely, a heavy reliance on motorised transportation contributes to sedentary lifestyles, obesity rates, and consequent chronic diseases. By prioritizing active modes of transportation, such as cycling or walking, individuals can improve cardiovascular health while decreasing carbon emissions, showcasing the natural symbiosis between health promotion and environmental sustainability.

3.2. Environmental Actions for Health Promotion

Encouraging sustainable practices that promote health can trigger profound positive effects on both the individual's and the planet's well-being. Ranging from dietary changes to altering transport modes, there are countless opportunities for adopting beneficial, eco-friendly behaviors.

Promotion of plant-based diets offers a prime example of this correlation. Such diets are known to reduce cardiovascular diseases, improve gut health, and support weight management. Simultaneously, they demand less land and water and generate fewer greenhouse gases compared to diets rich in animal products.

To further emphasize this, the cultivation of vegetables requires significantly less water and land than needed to raise livestock. A plant-based diet thus reduces strain on earth's resources while fostering personal health improvement.

3.3. From Awareness to Action

For many, the link between individual health and the well-being of our environment seems rather abstract, but the causal relationships are increasingly well-documented. An essential step for health promotion, then, is creating awareness of this connection.

The necessity of sustainable actions for health escalates manifold during crises like pandemics and climate emergencies. For instance, amidst the COVID-19 pandemic, environmental changes became more apparent as human activities dwindled, pointing towards the immense impact of human behavior.

Educational and awareness programs are crucial for communicating the importance of the role we play in impacting the environment and, subsequently, our health. Therefore, awareness translates to proactive action, with initiatives like community-based gardens or local cleanup events gaining momentum.

3.4. The Role of Policy and Concomitant Efforts

Government policies can powerfully affect individual and community behaviors concerning health and sustainability. From nationwide initiatives that encourage recycling or banning single-use plastic to local urban planning that favours pedestrian-friendly environments and green spaces, policies can play a substantial role in fostering sustainability and promoting health.

However, these steps are most effective when combined with individual efforts to make environmentally-friendly choices in daily life. No policy can match the collective impact of millions of people consciously shifting towards a more sustainable and healthier way of living.

3.5. The Rewards of Embracing Sustainable Fitness

There's no doubt that the pursuit of sustainable fitness can significantly enhance our sense of well-being. As we work to improve our health, we can simultaneously contribute towards healing the planet. These twin goals are not only compatible but symbiotic.

Practices such as outdoor fitness activities, active commuting (like walking or cycling), or incorporating locally sourced, organic foods rich in nutrients into the daily diet can yield an immediate positive impact on personal fitness, environment, and community health.

3.6. In Conclusion

Sustainability and health are profoundly interconnected. As we move towards a more sustainable lifestyle, we contribute to our health and the health of the planet. From the food we consume to how we commute and work out, our choices matter. With awareness and collective action, we can attain our fitness goals while also contributing to rejuvenating the earth. After all, there is no healthier choice than that which sustains both personal well-being and the health of our planet.

Chapter 4. Organic Living: Healthy You, Healthy Planet

The first step toward a sustainable lifestyle is understanding the concept of organic living. Largely, it means choosing products - food, cosmetics, clothes - that are grown or made naturally, without the use of harmful chemicals, preservatives, or genetically modified organisms (GMOs). Organic living does more than promote individual health; it contributes to environmental well-being, ultimately creating a ripple effect of benefits for our planet.

4.1. The Power of Organic Consumption

The foods we eat profoundly affect our health, especially over the long term. Consuming organic food, free of synthetic pesticides and insecticides, helps you avoid harmful substances often linked with severe health conditions. A review in the British Journal of Nutrition revealed that organic crops, on average, have higher concentrations of certain nutrients, such as antioxidants. Consuming these nutrient-dense foods can help ward off various lifestyle diseases.

Similarly, natural, chemical-free skin-care products tend to cause fewer skin irritations, allergies, and inflammation. Additionally, organic clothing, produced without toxic chemicals during cultivation and processing, is gentler on your skin and causes fewer allergic reactions.

Opting for organic food also makes a positive difference to the environment by reducing the chemical load. Organic farming practices nourish the soil, increase biodiversity, and help keep water resources clean, contributing to a healthier eco-system.

4.2. Organic Living: Beyond Your Plate

Embracing organic living goes beyond the food you consume. Here's how you can extend this practice:

1. **Household Products**: Choose cleaning products made of natural, non-toxic ingredients. Commercial cleaners usually contain harsh chemicals that are harmful to you and the environment. Plant-based, bio-degradable cleaners are an effective alternative.

2. **Gardening**: Grow your own organic fruits, vegetables, and herbs. This not only ensures you have fresh organically grown produce but also reduces your carbon footprint. Composting kitchen waste offers a rich nutrient source for your plants and decreases household waste.

3. **Clothing**: Opt for organic fabrics, made with natural fibers like cotton, hemp, or bamboo. These materials are grown and processed without harmful chemicals, making them healthier for you to wear and better for the planet.

4. **Skincare and Cosmetics**: Use products made with organic, chemical-free ingredients that are healthier for your skin. They're often packaged sustainably, too, reducing waste and pollution.

4.3. The Fitness Connection

Maintaining a regular and well-balanced fitness regimen directly benefits your physical health. But have you considered how it aligns with organic living? Organic food, packed with nutrients, fuels your body for exercise, while consuming enough water keeps you hydrated. Organically produced clothing, from your sports bra to your workout leggings, can help avoid skin irritations often associated with synthetic fabrics.

Additionally, consider outdoor workouts. Not only will this reduce energy consumption, but exposure to natural settings can boost mental health, improving motivation to exercise regularly.

4.4. Simple Swaps for a Sustainable Fitness Routine

1. **Ditch Plastic Bottles**: Replace single-use plastic water bottles with reusable metal or glass ones. They're more durable and safer, as they don't leach harmful chemicals.

2. **Eat Local and Seasonal Foods**: By doing so, you support local farmers, reduce carbon emissions associated with long-distance transport, and get the healthiest, tastiest foods.

3. **Choose Sustainable Fitness Gear**: From clothes to yoga mats, opt for sustainably made products whenever possible.

4. **Try Active Commuting**: Consider walking, cycling, or even running to your destination. It's a great way to incorporate daily activity while cutting down on carbon emissions.

4.5. Challenges and Solutions to Organic Living

Though beneficial, organic living comes with its set of challenges. Organic products are often more expensive due to costlier farming practices, less demand, and not being subsidized like conventional farming. Additionally, they may not be readily available, and their shelf life could be shorter because they lack preservatives.

Despite these challenges, there are ways to make organic living more practical:

1. **Start Small**: Begin with easily accessible, reasonably priced

organic products and gradually expand your organic purchases.

2. **Buy in Bulk**: Purchasing organic items in bulk can make them more cost-effective.

3. **Seasonal Shopping**: Choose seasonal organic produce. They're generally cheaper and fresher.

4. **Community Supported Agriculture (CSA) Programs**: Participating in CSA programs can connect you to local farmers for fresh, organic produce directly.

Organic living and physical fitness form a powerful duo that can dramatically upgrade your health while protecting the planet. Every organic choice you make creates a positive ripple effect, and every step, jog, or yoga pose performed in conscious alignment with sustainable values strengthens the bond between fitness and sustainability. Embrace the organic lifestyle, couple it with a sustainable fitness practice, and you'll be contributing to a healthier you and a greener Earth.

Chapter 5. Eco-Friendly Exercise: The Rising Trend

The environmental impact of our daily lives has become an increasing concern over the last few decades. As individuals take more responsibility for their carbon footprint, we've seen a growing trend towards eco-friendly exercises. If you're environmentally conscious and want to minimize your ecological impact while staying in top shape, these fitness practices can help you achieve just that.

5.1. The Concept of Eco-Friendly Exercise

Eco-friendly exercise incorporates physical activities that aim to decrease harm to the environment as much as possible. Simply put, it combines the goals of health and environmental impact lowering into a shared pursuit. This can involve fitness regimes that utilize minimal equipment, outdoor settings, or recycling initiatives. However, there's a broader philosophical shift at play here. The idea at the heart of eco-friendly exercise is dovetailing personal health with planetary health. In this way, the pursuit of fitness becomes a chance to protect and sustain the earth.

5.2. Reaping Dual Benefits

The benefits are twofold: not only does eco-friendly exercise contribute to physical health, but it also encourages a more sustainable lifestyle. Regular physical activity improves cardiovascular health and reduces the risk of various diseases. Simultaneously, eco-friendly exercise leads to a lower environmental impact and more responsible use of resources. This synergy has bred a fitness revolution where private health advances do not come at the environment's cost.

5.3. Trends in Eco-Friendly Exercise

As this concept gains traction, several sub-trends have emerged supporting it. Each one offers its unique mix of physical activity and environmental stewardship.

5.3.1. Outdoor Workouts

With the rise of eco-friendly exercise, gym-goers are returning to the great outdoors. Natural elements like hills, trees, and bodies of water offer the same resistance training, cardio, and flexibility workouts provided by traditional gym machinery, with zero carbon emissions. Outdoor workouts solely depend on the natural environments, thus leaving almost no carbon footprint. Whether it's trail running, park-based high-intensity interval training (HIIT) workouts, or swimming in natural bodies of water, outdoor workouts present an excellent eco-friendly exercise solution.

5.3.2. Green Gyms

Many gyms are adopting more sustainable practices to cater to environmentally conscious individuals. These "green gyms" power their facilities with renewable energy, install energy-efficient equipment, and encourage reduced water usage. Some innovative gyms even harness the kinetic energy generated by cardio equipment like treadmills and convert it back into electrical power. This form of energy recycling significantly reduces the gym establishments' overall carbon footprint.

5.3.3. Yoga and Pilates

Traditional practices like yoga and pilates are making a comeback due to their minimal environmental impact. They typically require little to no machinery—just a mat—and can be performed nearly anywhere. These practices not only emphasize mindfulness, flexibility, and strength but also encourage an environmental consciousness.

5.3.4. Plogging

The Swedish have merged fitness and environmental care into a new phenomenon called plogging—picking up litter while jogging. Individuals or groups run with a bag or pail, collecting any litter they encounter on their route. This act of environmental stewardship doubles as light resistance training, making it a comprehensive workout. The practice has taken off globally, as people appreciate how it combines an outdoor workout with tangible environmental action.

5.4. The Role of Technology in Eco-Friendly Exercise

In a world where consumers demand transparency, many fitness apps capitalize on the growing eco-consciousness, offering ways to track and offset their carbon footprint. These innovative solutions foster a strong link between individual wellness and global sustainability. Some apps provide opportunities to donate to environmental charities per mile run, or they track the emissions saved by choosing cycling or walking over a car ride, and so on. By integrating sustainability into these technological platforms, achieving fitness goals will also mean making substantial contributions to environmental preservation.

5.5. On the Path to Sustainability

By adopting eco-friendly exercise, every individual can help reduce the strain on our planet while improving their physical health. It's a win-win situation for both the individual and the environment. The rising trend of sustainable fitness practices is an encouraging sign of increased environmental awareness among the general public. As we continue to evolve in our approach to exercise, we hope to see more innovations that allow us to break a sweat without breaking our planet.

By embodying the practices discussed in this chapter, you'll be well on your way to Sustainable Fitness, a fitness regimen that respects both your health and the health of our planet. It's your chance to reap the benefits of exercise while playing your part in a more sustainable world. And remember that the goal isn't just to change your workout—it's to change your mindset. In this way, Sustainable Fitness will resonate far beyond the gym or the hiking trail into every aspect of your life, including your diet, your commute, and even your buying habits.

So go ahead, lace up those sneakers, and embark on a fitness journey that contributes to a healthier, greener world. You may be just one person, but when it comes to preserving the planet, every step counts.

Chapter 6. Understanding the Carbon Footprint of Your Workout

The carbon footprint of our daily routines and activities, including our workout regimen, plays a vital role in defining our environment. By understanding it, we can find ways to reduce our emissions and sync our fitness with sustainability goals.

6.1. Carbon Footprint: A Brief Overview

The term 'carbon footprint' refers to the total greenhouse gas emissions produced by a single entity, be it an individual, establishment, or a particular activity. Most often, it's measured in tons of carbon dioxide (CO_2) or CO_2 equivalents, which is a unit that converts the effect of different types of greenhouse gases, like methane, to an equivalent amount of CO_2. Although we don't usually see or think about these emissions, they're inextricably connected to almost everything we do. Therefore, to make our exercise regimen more sustainable, we first need to identify the areas where it contributes to our carbon footprint.

6.2. The Hidden Carbon Costs of Exercise

If you're a regular gym-goer, have you ever considered how the energy consumed by your favorite fitness center impacts the environment? From powering the various machines and lighting the space to heating, cooling, and even cleaning, every aspect of a gym's operation contributes to its carbon footprint. By extension, your workouts also contribute to this footprint.

Similarly, driving to the gym, running on asphalt, or producing your fitness equipment can also have significant carbon footprints. Even the clothes we wear when exercising, produced often from synthetic, petroleum-based fibers, have their carbon costs. When we consider these aspects, we realize that the carbon footprint of our workout regimen is more comprehensive than we initially thought.

6.3. Measuring the Carbon Footprint of Your Workout

Now that we understand how our workout can contribute to global carbon emissions, let's explore how to estimate this impact. The bad news is that accurate measurement is complex since it involves numerous variables, such as the energy efficiency of your gym or the fuel efficiency of your car. However, online tools and calculators can provide approximations.

One such tool is the Carbon Footprint Calculator, which allows you to calculate emissions from your car journeys. You can enter your vehicle's make and model, the type of fuel it uses, and your average miles per day to get an estimate. Another one is the Electricity Emissions Calculator, enabling you to calculate carbon emissions based on your electricity consumption. Remember, these are rough estimates, but they can give you some idea of the amount of CO2 related to your fitness activity.

6.4. Strategies to Minimize Your Workout's Carbon Footprint

Even though the carbon footprint from our fitness activities contributes to climate change, it's crucial to remember that exercise is essential for our health. The trick lies in finding balance and making our workouts more environmentally friendly. Here are some strategies that can help:

1. Walking or Cycling: If possible, replace driving with walking or cycling to your training location. Not only does it save on fuel and emissions, it's also a great workout.

2. Outdoor Exercise: Opt for outdoor workouts whenever possible. Activities like running, cycling, swimming, or hiking in nature require no electricity and hence have a smaller carbon footprint.

3. Sustainable Fitness Gear: Choosing ethical fitness gear made from sustainable materials can also make a significant difference.

4. Energy-Efficient Gym: If you must go to the gym, find one that uses renewable energy or adopts energy-saving measures.

By integrating these habits, we can make our workout routines more sustainable without compromising on our fitness goals.

6.5. In Conclusion

Your workout routine's carbon footprint is an integral part of your overall environmental impact. By understanding it and making conscious choices, we have the power to lessen our contribution to greenhouse gas emissions. By addressing the intersection of fitness and sustainability, we contribute to a healthier planet that can support our endeavors for a healthy body. This is a commitment to not just personal wellness but global wellness, presently and for the generations to come.

Chapter 7. Green Spaces for Active Places: The Power of Outdoor Exercise

Outdoor exercise carries dual benefits when done correctly: it promotes improved physical well-being and lends hand in preserving the delicate balance of the environment. It's not hard to envisage how path-free trails running through emerald woods, or hiking up a panoramic mountain appeals more to the senses than sweating it out inside a square box of walls. The fresh air outside, the sunlight against the skin, and the stimulating variation of the natural terrain provide a holistic workout experience - something not quite replicable within the four walls of a gym.

7.1. Benefits of Outdoor Exercise

Engaging with the outdoors, in pursuit of fitness, offers a unique blend of benefits. Physical exercise in the fresh air can uplift your mood significantly. Sunlight is an excellent source of vitamin D, essential for bone health and immunity. Walking on an uneven path helps improve balance and co-ordination while fresh air has a calming effect on the mind.

Furthermore, it has been reported that an outdoor environment can reduce cortisol, the stress hormone, more effectively than an indoor environment. The natural landscapes are said to provide a sense of peace that can lessen anxiety and depression, contributing to mental well-being in addition to physical fitness.

Another advantage is that outdoor activities involve little to no energy consumption from non-renewable sources compared to gyms which run on electricity. Be it powering the treadmills, lighting, air conditioning, or blaring music – it all adds up to a significant carbon footprint. Outdoor exercise, on the other hand, uses what the nature offers – gravity, body weight, natural elements – and thus is more eco-friendly.

7.2. Creating Green Spaces for Physical Activity

A direct way to promote outdoor exercise and reiterate its benefits is to create more green spaces or parks in our neighborhoods. These spaces not only provide a pleasant environment for physical activity, but also work as carbon sinks, reducing the amount of CO2 in the atmosphere. They act as the lungs of our cities, supplying fresh air while creating a setting for people to interact with nature.

However, creating these spaces isn't as straightforward as it sounds. It involves careful planning, adequate investment, and community participation. Land needs to be identified and then cleared without disturbing the ecosystem significantly. The inclusion of elements like trails, bike lanes, open spaces for yoga or Tai Chi, and adequate sitting arrangements should be considered. It should be ensured that these parks are accessible to all sections of society without any discrimination.

7.3. Participatory Urban Planning: A Key to Green Spaces

Participatory urban planning plays a crucial role here as it involves the local community in decision-making processes, thereby ensuring their needs and views are incorporated. Be it deciding the location of the park or the amenities to be included within – having input from people who would actually use the space can significantly boost its effectiveness and popularity.

Regular maintenance of these spaces is another aspect needing attention. Protection from defacement, ensuring cleanliness and safety are fundamentals of park management. Regular events like community clean-up drives or tree plantation drives can ensure people feel connected to their local green spaces, making it a shared responsibility.

7.4. City Forests and Green Roofs

Another concept gaining momentum is that of Urban Forestry or the creation of 'City Forests'. These involve the conversion of unused urban land into patches of forests using native species of plants. The forests act as green lungs, recreation centers, and can also host outdoor fitness classes, encouraging people to stay fit while connecting to nature.

Green Roofs, where the roofs of buildings are covered with vegetation, can also be developed as workout spots. Especially in densely developed urban areas where land is at a premium, converting roof tops into green spaces for physical activity can be a smart solution. Not only will it provide a place for exercise, but it also helps in improving the building's insulation, absorbing rainwater, and even acting as a small-scale habitat for birds.

7.5. Green Exercise Activism

Campaign building and community organization can significantly boost the popularity of outdoor exercise. Green exercise groups can be formed within communities that regularly organize outdoor fitness activities. These may include anything from simple walks in the park to more organized events like Bootcamp in the Park.

Fitness instructors can host regular workout sessions in green spaces, and events like 'Yoga Under The Tree' or 'Zumba in the Park' can become regular features. Such activities will not only encourage people to contribute to the conservation of these spaces but will also help in building a strong community ethos around the idea of sustainable fitness.

In conclusion, Outdoor Exercise is an essential constituent of Sustainable Fitness. It uses minimal resources while offering maximum benefits: physical, mental, and environmental. By making concerted community efforts and using innovative ideas to create and maintain green spaces, we contribute to a future where fitness routines are eco-friendly, providing benefits not just to individuals but also the planet. Through this harmonious blend, we can ensure a healthier us in a greener world.

Chapter 8. Sustainable Diet: Nutrition that Nourishes Both Body and Earth

In the quagmire of health and fitness, diet stands as an undisputed pillar. Yet, our nourishment habits have consequences not only for our bodies but also for the Earth. So, where do we find the right balance that can nourish our bodies and the planet? With challenge comes opportunity: the opportunity to craft a sustainable diet.

8.1. Understanding a Sustainable Diet

Within a sustainable diet, nutrition and environmental protection interweave, fostering a relationship of mutual growth. In technical terms, the Food and Agriculture Organization (FAO) defines a sustainable diet as one with "low environmental impacts which contribute to food and nutrition security and to healthy life for present and future generations."

But what does this mean for individuals? Firstly, it calls for a considerable reduction in meat and dairy consumption and a shift towards plant-based foods, while limiting the intake of processed and packaged food. These changes not only reduce health risks but also mitigate adverse environmental issues like greenhouse gas emissions, deforestation, and water pollution.

8.1.1. Health Benefits of a Plant-Based Diet

Going plant-based has been associated with numerous health benefits. Packed with fiber, antioxidants, and other nutrients, plant-based foods can help reduce the risk of chronic illnesses, like heart disease, type 2 diabetes, and certain cancers. According to studies, vegans also tend to have lower body mass indexes (BMIs), lower cholesterol and blood pressure levels, and a lower risk of death from heart disease. Quite simply, a well-planned plant-based diet can be incredibly beneficial for our long-term health.

8.1.2. Environmental Impacts of Animal Agriculture

On the environmental front, the excessive consumption of meat and dairy contributes significantly to climate change. Animal agriculture is, in fact, responsible for more greenhouse gas emissions than all the world's transportation systems combined. This is because of the methane production from ruminant animals like cows, land usage for growing animal feed, and deforestation for grazing lands. A sustainable diet thus involves lowering our consumption of these high-impact foods.

8.2. How to Adopt a Sustainable Diet

Adopting a sustainable diet doesn't have to imply radical alterations or sacrifices in taste and enjoyment. Many small shifts can make your dietary habits more eco-friendly and health-oriented.

8.2.1. Eat More Plant-Based Foods

Start by incorporating more fruits, vegetables, whole grains, legumes, nuts, and seeds into your diet. These foods are nutrient-dense and high in fiber, leading to satiety, optimal digestion, and overall good health. You don't have to completely give up on meat. Consider adopting a 'flexitarian' approach, where you prioritize plant-based meals but still indulge in meat and dairy occasionally.

8.2.2. Buy Local and Seasonal Produce

Eating seasonal produce is easier on the environment as it requires fewer resources to grow and transport. Moreover, it could be more nutritious and taste better, as it is harvested at peak ripeness. Local farmers markets are an excellent source for seasonal fruits and vegetables, and you'll be supporting your community simultaneously.

8.2.3. Minimize Processed Foods

Processed and packaged foods tend to be nutritionally inferior and often packed with unhealthy additives. Furthermore, their production and packaging cause substantial environmental harm due to energy usage, greenhouse gas emissions, and waste. Thus, prioritizing whole foods can improve your diet's sustainability quotient significantly.

8.3. The Sustainability of Seafood

Seafood often comes up in conversations about sustainable diets. While it's true that fish and shellfish can be rich sources of lean protein, omega-3 fatty acids, and other nutrients, our demand for seafood is outpacing supply posing a threat to marine ecosystems. Hence, we need to be mindful and choose sustainably sourced seafood. Look for labels such as the Marine Stewardship Council (MSC) to ensure the seafood you're buying is responsibly caught.

8.4. Conclusion

Transitioning to a sustainable diet is not only a personal health journey but also demonstrates compassion and responsibility towards our planet. This adoption is not about perfection; it's about making more conscious choices more often. As we understand the weight of our dietary choices, we fine-tune our food habits to a healthier rhythm, contributing to a symphony in sync with the

Earth's needs. Remember, every small change can have a big impact when gathered on a global scale.

In the pursuit of a healthier self and a greener Earth, a sustainable diet provides a path that caters to both. It's high time we realize – the health of the planet and our health are not separate; they are interconnected. As we provide our bodies with the proper nourishment it deserves, let's also strive to sustain the Earth, which serves as our home.

Chapter 9. Looking Beyond Plastic: Eco-Friendly Fitness Gear and Apparel

Our daily lives are intimately tied to plastic. It's in our homes, our workplaces, and, yes, even in our gyms. From our hydration bottles to our shin-comforting yoga mats, synthetic materials, especially plastic, abound in our fitness regimes. But, as we strive to become physically fit and healthy, could we also consider the health of the planet? That is the question at the center of our exploration in this section.

9.1. Rethinking Plastic: The Detrimental Impacts and the Need for Change

It's no secret that plastic pollution is a pressing environmental issue, with millions of tons ending up in our oceans every year. But why is this a problem? Well, plastic is not biodegradable. Instead, it breaks down into smaller pieces, or microplastics, that hotwire into the ecosystem, posing a significant threat to marine life and birds. Through the food web, these particles can also make their way into our bodies, with potential adverse health effects.

Our workout gear and apparel significantly contribute to this plastic problem. Synthetic materials such as polyester and nylon, both types of plastic, dominate this industry. While these fabrics offer strength, durability, and moisture-wicking properties, we cannot ignore their environmental impact. Releasing microplastics into our water systems with every wash, these textiles have unforeseen consequences for our earth's ecosystems and our bodies.

In this context, the need for eco-friendly fitness gear and apparel is not a frill but a demand of the times. Fortunately, many brands are responding to this call, developing products that are not only high-performing but also tread lightly on the environment.

9.2. Rising Tide of Eco-conscious Brands

Enter a new generation of fitness brands, committed to sustainable practices in every aspect of their operations. These pioneers in the industry are challenging norms, innovating product design, and setting a new standard in environmental consciousness.

For instance, take Adidas, which in collaboration with Parley for the Oceans, has created shoes and clothes from recycled ocean plastic. Then there's Girlfriend Collective, which transforms old water bottles, fishing nets, and other waste into chic, sustainable activewear. Manduka, too, offers eco-friendly yoga mats, props, and towels made from natural or recycled materials.

Actively engaging in responsible sourcing, ethical production practices, and transparency in operations, these brands are making it easier for us to choose fitness gear and apparel that aligns with our environmental values.

9.3. Guide to Choosing Eco-Friendly Fitness Gear and Apparel

Finding more sustainable alternatives to conventional plastic-heavy fitness products can be a daunting task, especially with the myriad options on the market. This guide will help you make better, more informed choices.

1. **Material Considerations:** Look for naturally sourced or recycled

materials. Cotton, hemp, bamboo, and wool are great alternatives to synthetic textiles. Some companies also use innovative materials like eucalyptus pulp or recycled fishing nets. Check the product labels to ensure the claims are genuine.

2. **Production Process:** A product's environmental impact isn't only about the materials used but also how it's made. For instance, is the production process water-intensive? Does it result in greenhouse gas emissions? Companies that are transparent about their production processes usually have less to hide.

3. **Company Practices:** Do they engage in ethical labor practices? Do they prioritize energy-efficient operations? Do they participate in any recycling or take-back programs? Companies with comprehensive eco-friendly practices are generally a better choice.

4. **Product Lifespan:** High-quality, durable gear may be more expensive, but it'll last longer and have less of an environmental impact in the long run.

5. **End of Life:** Consider what will happen to your gear when it's no longer usable. Can it be recycled, or will it end up in a landfill?

9.4. Caring for Your Gear to Extend its Lifespan

Once you have your eco-friendly gear, how you maintain it significantly impacts its lifespan and ongoing environmental footprint. Here are some tips to help you care for your gear:

1. **Washing less often:** Fabrics made from natural fibers or recycled materials may not require frequent washes. Overwashing can degrade the material and shorten its lifespan.

2. **Cold wash:** Washing your gear in cold water not only saves energy but also helps maintain the fabric integrity, especially for synthetics.

3. **Air dry:** Whenever possible, skip the dryer and air-dry your gear. It's better for them and the planet.

4. **Repairing:** If your gear gets a small tear, don't throw it away. Repair it. Many companies even offer repair services for their products.

9.5. The Road Ahead

As we march towards a sustainable future, eco-friendly fitness gear and apparel serve as powerful symbols of change, reminding us that every choice we make has an impact. Here, the fitness industry exemplifies this shift, pointing the way toward a healthier planet.

While adopting sustainable fitness gear doesn't negate the environmental challenges humanity faces, it's a step in the right direction. A small step, to be sure, but as we know, our fitness journeys are made up of countless small steps, each one taking us closer to our health goals. As we pursue this journey, let us be reminded that health isn't merely personal—it's global, too.

With thoughtful choices in fitness gear and apparel, we can give the planet a breather, literally and figuratively. Each sustainable purchase, use, and disposal is a vote for a healthier planet. As the saying goes: "We do not inherit the Earth from our ancestors—we borrow it from our children."

So, as we sweat it out in the gym or hit the road for that early morning jog, let's not just do it for ourselves. Let's do it also in the spirit of planetary stewardship, bearing in mind that our health is deeply intertwined with the health of the planet.

Chapter 10. Activism through Fitness: Using Sports for Environmental Advocacy

The amplification of environmental issues through sports isn't a new phenomenon. Athletes, sports teams, and even entire sporting events have been leveraging their platforms to bring awareness to environmental sustainability. But it's not just about awareness; it's about driving action.

10.1. Athletes as Environmental Advocates

In the world of sports, athletes are more than just competitors; they are influencers, role models, and trendsetters. With their reach extending far beyond the realm of their sport, they have the power to influence the perspectives and actions of millions across the globe.

One stellar example of an athlete-turned-environmental advocate is Lewis Pugh. A long-distance swimmer and United Nations Patron of the Oceans, Pugh uses his sporting achievements to promote ocean conservation. By swimming in some of the world's most endangered and challenging ecosystems, he highlights the direct impacts of climate change on these regions and advocates for their protection.

Similarly, professional snowboarder Jeremy Jones founded Protect Our Winters (POW), an organization dedicated to educating and mobilizing the winter sports community to lead the fight against climate change. These athletes exemplify how one can engage in fitness while championing environmental causes, effectively uniting their passion for sports with their commitment to sustainability.

10.2. Sports Teams and Leagues Prioritizing Sustainability

It's not only individual athletes who are leveraging the platform of sports for environmental advocacy. Sports teams and entire leagues have taken notable strides in promoting sustainable practices.

The Philadelphia Eagles' "Go Green" initiative is an industry-leading approach to environmental sustainability. The National Football League (NFL) team powers their stadium with renewable energy and has implemented an extensive recycling program. Further, they work to offset their carbon emissions by planting trees.

Even at larger scales, sports organizations like the National Basketball Association (NBA) and the Union of European Football Associations (UEFA) have integrated sustainability into their operations. They promote the use of renewable energy, encourage recycling at their events, and work to offset carbon emissions resulting from their activities.

These examples demonstrate how sports entities of all sizes can utilize their influence to promote environmental responsibility.

10.3. Utilising Mega Sporting Events

Mega sporting events like the Olympic Games and FIFA World Cup offer a unique opportunity to promote environmental awareness and sustainable practices. These events garner attention from billions worldwide, turning the global spotlight onto the host cities and their environmental initiatives.

The 2016 Rio Olympic Games were a milestone in sustainable event planning, as organizers implemented a comprehensive sustainability management plan. This included measures for waste management, biodiversity protection, and carbon offsetting initiatives. Similarly, the FIFA World Cup in Qatar 2022 aims to be the first carbon-neutral World Cup, investing in projects to offset its carbon emissions.

However, these events also generate critics highlighting the massive environmental footprint left behind. It calls for organizers and participants alike to reflect on the true sustainability of these occasions.

10.4. Local Communities and Grassroot Movements

At the root of global change are local actions. Grassroots movements that combine sports and environmental activism have a crucial role in driving sustainable behaviors and policy changes within their communities.

Community run clubs and sports leagues are starting to recognize the importance of sustainability. Not only are they incorporating local environmental issues into their events and programs but also safeguarding the natural environments often required for their activities.

These local organizations range from recreational clubs to competitive teams, all incorporating environmental advocacy into their activities. Be it through beach clean-ups after a local surfing contest or tree planting initiatives by hiking clubs — their combined effort creates a significant impact.

10.5. The Pathway Forward

Essentially, integrating environmental advocacy into sports is about fostering a culture of sustainability within the athletic community. It entails educating athletes, teams, and fans about environmental issues, inspiring them to make sustainable choices, and empowering them to advocate for environmental protection.

A healthy planet is the backbone of our health and fitness journey. Through sports, we have the opportunity to echo the importance of this truth to millions of individuals worldwide. By weaving environmental advocacy into the fabric of our fitness pursuits, we can help to ensure the longevity of our planet, along with our own health and wellbeing.

It begins with us — each sweat-drenched training session, each local sports event attended or organized, each green choice made — they all culminate in a broader narrative of sustainable fitness. After all, our ultimate goal is not just to improve ourselves but the planet that enables our improvement. As we move forward, let our mantra be: In fitness and in health, for us and for the Earth.

Chapter 11. Cultivating a Sustainable Fitness Lifestyle: Methodologies and Inspirations

The quest for individual fitness and health goes hand in hand with preserving our planet. In cultivating a sustainable fitness lifestyle, it's important to understand that personal behavior and habits significantly contribute to the state of the environment. Routine actions, like the mode of travel to the gym, the type of diet kept, and the habit of recycling, play a crucial role in defining the relationship between fitness and sustainability. This chapter seeks to inspire and educate on methodologies for cultivating a sustainable fitness lifestyle.

11.1. Adopt a Green Gym Routine

Our means of getting around heavily contribute to environmental pollution. Visit any fitness facility near peak hours and you'll likely find a packed parking lot. Many gym-goers default to their cars, oblivious of the significant carbon emission their trips entail.

Rather than driving, consider walking, running, or biking to the gym. These modes of transportation serve as a warm-up, require no fuel, and produce zero emissions. For those who live far from the fitness facility, carpools or public transportation offer more sustainable options.

Additionally, explore the idea of outdoor workouts. Not only does this reduce energy usage required for indoor gym operations, it offers a refreshing change in scenery.

To engage in a sustainable fitness lifestyle is to go beyond personal advantage. Patronize fitness facilities that emphasize green strategies. These may include solar power, recycled rubber flooring, and equipment that generates electricity.

11.2. Eco-friendly Exercise Gear

Exercise gear contributes a significant amount to landfill waste worldwide. Non-biodegradable items, such as sport shoes, yoga mats, and workout attire, take years to decompose. Therefore, purchasing eco-friendly fitness gear becomes essential in cultivating a sustainable fitness lifestyle.

Select exercise clothes made with sustainable materials like organic cotton or bamboo. These materials have lower environmental impacts in farming and manufacturing.

As for sport shoes, numerous brands have turned to more sustainable means of production, employing recycled materials and minimizing waste. Furthermore, instead of disposing of your old shoes, consider recycling them.

Additionally, keep a reusable water bottle handy for hydration instead of buying single-use plastic bottles. These day-to-day choices influence the demand and production of single-use plastic items, and picking reusable alternatives can have a significant impact.

11.3. Adopt Plant-based Diets

Diet plays a crucial role in both personal fitness and sustainability. Livestock farming accounts for a substantial amount of greenhouse gas emissions and water usage. Shifting to a plant-based diet can significantly reduce your carbon footprint.

Plant-based diets are rich in fiber, vitamins, and minerals, proving beneficial for weight management and overall health. Research indicates that plant-based eating can prevent certain diseases and improve longevity.

Transitioning to a plant-friendly diet doesn't need to be abrupt. Begin with a few meat-free days a week and gradually increase the number of plant-based meals.

11.4. Sustainability-focused Fitness Goals

The top-down approach to cultivating a sustainable fitness lifestyle involves setting sustainability-focused fitness goals. These goals revolve around two aspects: individual fitness and contribution to environmental preservation. For instance, setting a goal to walk or cycle to work not only benefits personal health but also significantly reduces carbon emissions.

To measure the impact of your actions, consider carbon calculators, which roughly estimate individual carbon footprints based on personal habits and lifestyle. Use these insights to assess your contribution to greenhouse gas emissions and set targets for reduction.

11.5. The Influence of Mindset

Achieving a sustainable fitness lifestyle requires a significant mindset shift. It demands seeing beyond narrow fitness goals to larger sustainability issues.

Regular mindfulness practices can help cultivate this broader perspective. Mindfulness involves being fully present and consciously making decisions that support personal and planetary health. Journaling is a valuable tool for nurturing mindfulness, helping to track both fitness journey and sustainability efforts.

In conclusion, cultivating a sustainable fitness lifestyle requires deliberate effort and understanding that individual habits significantly contribute to the state of our environment. By adopting green gym routines, using eco-friendly gear, shifting towards plant-based diets, setting sustainability-focused fitness goals, and adopting a conscious mindset, fitness enthusiasts can contribute significantly towards a healthier, greener world.

Remember, the journey towards a sustainable fitness lifestyle is not a sprint. It's a marathon. Adopt changes at a comfortable pace, celebrate small victories and stay consistent. With time, these efforts will reap both personal and planetary rewards.